NUTRITION

FOR

REPRODUCTION

A detailed guide on diets that
increase pregnancy chances

Owen D. Spark

TABLE OF CONTENT

INTRODUCTION

As people become increasingly conscious of global warming and the need to live more ecologically responsible lifestyles, they are adding locally grown organic food to their meals. Organic farmers employ natural techniques to saturate their soil and manage pests rather than synthetic pesticides, resulting in vegetable plants that are stronger, healthier, and, for many consumers, even tastier.

Anyone learning to cook requires recipes they can follow to prepare nutritious meals, and if those meals include organic ingredients, having one or more organic recipe books may make making delightful side dishes and main courses much easier. Anyone using organic ingredients in conventional recipes may discover that they need to adjust the recipes to take into account the richer flavors.

Following fertility, diet is really simple and doesn't require much time. To ascertain whether you have any deficiencies that should be corrected first, It's one of the simplest ways to look after your health and provide your body the nutrition you and your unborn kid may need. After your body is healthy and the fertility diet starts to function, you'll be well on your way to a healthy and successful pregnancy.

Nutritionists have been urging us to adopt healthy lifestyles and change our eating habits for decades. We all need a strong rationale to cease indulging in unhealthy activities since, in reality, we are all irresponsible when it comes to our diets.

On the other hand, when a certain health condition manifests, it prompts us to consider life more than anything else. We would be willing to completely alter our habits if the doctor recommended it. One of the key reasons why some couples find it difficult to achieve long-lasting contentment in this situation is infertility concerns.

You can learn that your capacity to conceive, whether you're a woman or a guy, can be significantly impacted by the food you eat by picking up any random book on a fertility diet. Certain meals can support the proper operation of our body while others might harm it. People who wish to start a family but haven't had the chance to conceive yet would do well to start with the guidance that follows. By incorporating them into a sensible fertility diet plan, you can raise your chances of getting pregnant.

CHAPTER ONE

ALTERNATIVES TO BOOST FERTILITY

We have identified different simple modifications that provide a significant increase in fertility for women with ovulation-related infertility. As follows:

Steer clear of trans fats, the artery-clogging fats that are included in a lot of commercially produced goods and fast meals.

Increase your consumption of unsaturated vegetable oils like canola or olive oil.

Consume more protein from vegetables, such as beans and nuts, and less from animal sources.

Opt for whole grains and other types of carbs rather than highly processed carbohydrates, which spike blood sugar and insulin fast. Whole grains and other sources of carbohydrates have lower, delayed impacts on blood sugar and insulin.

Have a modest serving of full-fat yogurt, ice cream, or skim milk every day; temporarily substitute full-fat versions of frozen yogurt, cottage cheese, and other dairy products for their low- or no-fat counterparts.

Take a vitamin supplement including folic acid and other B vitamins.

Consume lots of fruits, vegetables, legumes, and supplements; avoid red meat.

Beverages are important: water is fantastic, coffee, tea, and alcohol are OK in moderation, and sugary sodas should not be opened.

Work to maintain a healthy weight. Ovulation may be accelerated if you are overweight by decreasing between 5 and 10% of your body weight.

Start an everyday workout routine if you aren't already. Increase the intensity of your exercises if you currently exercise. Don't overdo it, however, particularly if you are already pretty slim since too much activity might harm conception.

Infertility is defined by medical texts as the circumstance when a couple is unable to produce a child even after a year of regular sexual activity and without using any kind of birth control.

The reasons for infertility are numerous:

Infertility in women: Infertile Women may experience:

- Age affects the ovulation process in women, which is an event where hormonal signals and physical occurrences are related.
- Cervical causes, in which the sperm is prevented from passing through the

uterus's mouth for a variety of reasons.

- Pelvic causes are those that have to do with anatomy and are brought on by any disturbance of the pelvic structure.

Men's Infertility: This may be brought on by issues with the genitalia, such as undeveloped testicles, infections, exposure to metals, and medicine (for instance, high blood pressure medication).

Regular causes

Infertility is also brought on by certain lifestyle choices, including the use of lubricants, infrequent intercourse, anorexia, stress, hunger, and extensive alcohol, cigarette, and drug usage. Then there are some more common variables, such as STDs, physical injuries, etc.

Approaches to boosting fertility

Between October and March, women attain their peak fertility, while between February and March, males produce the highest-quality sperm. That is the greatest time for conception, according to experts, so this is merely an observation of how nature works its magic on people.

Smoking is one of the factors that contribute to infertility because tobacco smoke includes chemicals that affect both men's and women's reproductive systems, including nicotine, carbon dioxide, and many more. To reduce the likelihood of becoming infertile, one must stop smoking.

The use of alcohol must be reduced since it reduces sperm count. Additionally, caffeine must be avoided since it affects both men's and women's fertility.

Stressful lifestyles should be avoided. Nowadays, both sexes live unbalanced lives while pursuing fame and wealth. They are under continual stress while working for their financial aspirations and business objectives. Stress lowers the immune system, harms the reproductive system, and has been linked to infertility in both men and women.

Wholesome eating. This is not to suggest that one should binge eat, but fasting and anorexia mess with sex hormones. And the same is true if food is consumed in excess.

So, consume the amount of food that is healthy for your body, as will be listed in this book.

Adopt a workout routine and follow it through. Exercise revs up the body's metabolic rate, fortifies the heart, and tones every organ. A couple should not deprive themselves of the best time of their lives by having a child by becoming infertile, which is mostly caused by the way men and women live their lives. Hopefully, the above-mentioned methods for boosting fertility will enable you to have the child of your dreams.

CHAPTER TWO

THINGS TO AVOID DOING TO BOOST FERTILITY

Numerous infertile couples are frantically looking for ways to increase their chances of conception, whether it be through their physicians, family, friends, the media, the internet, books, etc. However, there are several things I believe you should be aware of if you wish to conceive quickly.

We ought to discuss our way of life. Concerns about your future, your life, or even the possibility of becoming pregnant are unwarranted. Stress is very tough to become pregnant since it messes with your hormones. Depression may result, which compromises your fertility and makes becoming pregnant challenging.

You and your spouse need to learn to adapt and relax to increase fertility. As long as you engage in activities and tasks that make you happy and enhance your quality of life, activity and productivity may significantly lessen your stress.

The second biggest thing you need to stay away from is complacency. The greatest probability of success is with early therapy. Couples may reference their fertility charts when determining the best time to start trying for a child if there are indicators of impaired fertility.

Exist any foods you should steer clear of if you want to increase fertility?

- Overcooked meats
- Cooked eggs
- Refined white carbohydrates, particularly white flour

Pasteurized milk (which has been linked to infertility when consumed often), and these other foods should all be avoided if feasible. By ingesting 3-6 capsules of bee pollen daily, the production of sexual hormones in both men and women may be greatly boosted.

Add two raw egg yolks to a glass of carrot juice each day to get an organic lecithin boost that helps sperm grow robust. A prolonged tryptophan shortage is often the root cause of infertility in both men and women. Tryptophan, a crucial amino acid involved in nerve function, is abundant in bananas. For the growth of sperm and ovaries, wheat germ oil, which is high in organic vitamin E, should be consumed twice daily—after breakfast and supper. Celery, raw spinach, and raw fish are among other nourishing meals (sashimi).

When attempting to become pregnant, caffeine, alcohol, cigarettes, and other substances should be avoided (and while pregnant and breastfeeding). It is best to avoid these harmful substances. Environmental toxins like chemicals, radiation, opioids, heavy metal exposure, smoking, excessive alcohol consumption, drug use, and pollution can cause low sperm counts or poor sperm motility.

Female infertility is most commonly brought on by ovulatory issues, which have an impact on hormones, menstrual cycles, and conception. About 15% of these ailments are related to weight issues, namely being overweight or obese.

Furthermore, due to the increased estrogen levels linked to obesity, precancerous alterations in the uterus may often be reversed.

How should obesity be controlled?

When possible, stay away from meals that are especially heavy in sugar, saturated fat, or trans fat. Your diet should include whole grains, fruits, vegetables, lean sources of protein, and frequent exercise. Gastric bypass surgery may result in healthy weight loss even with just light kinds of exercise, such as walking or low-impact aerobics. Surgery is often used to decrease appetite in obese persons.

I'm hoping what I stated and advised against would boost your chances of becoming pregnant. I'm certain that with careful preparation, you may also have the opportunity to hold the healthiest kid in your arms.

What Role Does Diet Play in Conception?

There are several strategies to increase fertility, as well as a chance that taking certain meals and vitamins may help an infertility treatment work.

One of the meals to take for fertility is a multivitamin. Numerous studies have shown the benefits of multivitamins for improving fertility, especially for women who should take folic acid supplements. 400 mcg of folic acid per day is advised for females to help prevent brain and spinal cord birth abnormalities in fetuses. Prescription vitamins are not required; a variety of over-the-counter prenatal multivitamins are suitable.

However, you may be able to claim a multivitamin as a qualified item under your flexible spending account if your doctor does provide a prescription for one (i.e., an employer-sponsored account where an employee puts away a percentage of wages for tax-free health and medical expenses).

When possible, be sure to drink clean water. If you want to increase your chances of becoming pregnant, you must cut out artificial sweeteners and drinks, including diet sodas. As alternatives, think of flavored carbonated water or beverages sweetened with stevia, a natural plant extract. Although it is advised to drink 6 to 8 glasses of clean water daily, those with certain medical conditions should first see their physicians since they may need a modification of this advice to suit their particular requirements.

Neither diet nor processed foods should be consumed.

Eating "fake" meals won't completely reduce your chances of becoming pregnant, but they aren't fertility diet foods that support the reproductive system, improve fertility, or make infertility treatments more effective. One may limit or stay away from the following foods:

- The main aisles of your grocery store are where you may get processed goods that are often packed or boxed. Any food that has a health claim, including "low fat," "low cholesterol," or "No Trans Fat" sweets, juices, and sugary beverages.

- Artificial sweeteners like Equal, Splenda, Sweet'N Low, and other brands leave a white sugary residue on baked items, including loaves of bread, crackers, and muffins.

- Even the healthful cereal kinds found at health food stores have undergone processing.

- Tofurkey, Not-dogs, and other "fake" foods and meals are used as butter substitutes, such as margarine.

The production of endogenous hormones has been demonstrated to be disturbed by soy-based products, any product that includes high fructose corn syrup, partially hydrogenated oil, or artificial colors.

Consume foods that are most closely related to nature and behave as your forebears did.

Include the following food options in your diet for fertility:

It may seem frightening to those who have depended on diet foods to control their weight for years, but whole food products promote fertility and raise your chances of becoming pregnant. An example would be cooking eggs using real butter. Grass-fed, organic full-fat milk from cows or goats is preferable to skim or low-fat milk, which has powdered milk and oxidized cholesterol added.

Limit your consumption of grains to a small number since a significant amount is not necessary in your diet. The recommended grains include

- Lentils
- Beans
- Quinoa
- Brown rice
- Buckwheat

Eat unprocessed bread such as

- Gluten-free bread
- True sourdough bread, or
- Grains that have been sprouted.

When possible, eat organic food. Consuming organic foods has benefits for your fertility and overall health, despite the fact that they may be more expensive than non-organic foods and so may have a negative financial impact. If you don't have much money for organic food, try to eat as much of the following:

- Apples

- Bell peppers
- Celery
- Cherries
- Imported grapes
- Nectarines
- Peaches
- Pears
- Potatoes
- Red raspberries
- Spinach
- Strawberries

Additionally, it is believed that these foods are very pesticide-contaminated.

When it comes to produce, some of the least contaminated options are

- Asparagus
- Avocados
- Broccoli

- Bananas
- Cauliflower
- Kiwi
- Sweet corn
- Onions
- Mangos
- Papayas
- Pineapple
- Sweet peas

If an organic option is not available, these produce items may still be eaten as conventionally grown food.

Even if the packaging indicates that the food has already been cleaned, it is still advisable to wash any pre-packaged food, whether it is organic or not, to eliminate any possible contaminants.

Consume pasteurized chicken and beef that has only been fed grass, preferably organic, and that has not received any hormones throughout the rearing process.

The nutritional density of fish caught in the wild is higher than that of fish cultivated in aquaculture. Examples of large fish with a high mercury content include sharks, tilefish, and swordfish. The most that pregnant women should consume each week is 12 ounces of low-mercury fish. For instance, canned shrimp, pollock, and salmon.

Eliminating plastics is essential to a fertility diet. Studies have shown that the presence of BPA or bisphenol lowers fertility in both men and women. Put all plastic bottles and containers out of your house. Instead of buying "steam in the bag" vegetables, buy fresh vegetables and prepare them on the stovetop or in a steamer. Buy drinking vessels without BPA if possible.

Consider cleansing as a way to jump-start your diet for fertility. Getting rid of organic contaminants and preparing your body for fertility treatments and delivery may both be accomplished via detoxification, which is another word for cleansing. Many programs are available on the market. Choose a routine that includes entire, organic, and unprocessed meals as well as supplements manufactured from whole foods.

CHAPTER THREE

INCREASING FERTILITY NATURALLY

One in seven couples has trouble getting pregnant because of poor health. Our bodies frequently forbid us from being pregnant until we have repaired our physical and mental wellness. If we have a healthy, balanced diet, we can regenerate and repair, which will help us have a healthy pregnancy. On numerous occasions, a high intake of processed and refined foods, as well as environmental toxins, are to blame for our bodies' nutritional deficiencies. Studies have indicated that maintaining a healthy diet and lifestyle increases the likelihood of conception.

Traditional Chinese Medicine has used nutrition for thousands of years to enhance and rebalance the body and hormones to achieve the best possible reproductive harmony and wellness. Fertility can be increased by the use of herbs, acupuncture, and a healthy lifestyle. The secret to success is to treat your body as though you are already pregnant by following a natural fertility diet and staying away from anything that could harm a developing fetus.

A dietary regimen known as a "fertility diet" is designed to assist your body to readjust so you can overcome any fertility issues you may be dealing with. It is an eating pattern that supports the body's reproductive functions by ingesting foods rich in specific nutrients and minerals required for hormone production and balance, healthy egg development, strong sperm in males, and many other benefits.

Adopting a fertility diet to boost fertility and prepare your body for pregnancy is one of the most significant decisions you can make. Your body and mind will both gain from it. Consuming a nutritious diet is one more step you may take to manage your fertility. Many studies have shown that certain dietary changes can increase the likelihood of ovulation, lower the risk of recurrent miscarriages, rebalance hormones, and support a healthy pregnancy. Since food contains the building blocks for hormones, nutrition is crucial for sustaining a healthy body and reproductive system. Antioxidants included in food are essential for protecting the egg against the harm caused by free radicals.

Your diet now will have an impact on the quality of your eggs in 90 days. Anyone can adhere to a fertility diet, regardless of their location, age, financial condition, time limits, or fertility difficulties. We all need to eat, therefore start eating in a way that supports fertility.

Studies show that a slow-carb, primarily plant-based diet greatly increases fertility. The foundation of a healthy diet has long been emphasized in eastern medicine to be whole, organic meals made from plants.

Sweet potatoes, garlic are proven to increase fertility other foods include:

- Tofu
- Soybeans
- Kelp
- Green leafy vegetables
- Pumpkin seeds
- Sunflower seeds
- Strawberries
- Peaches
- Raisins
- Olive oil
- Whey protein
- Oats
- Brown rice

- Barley
- Wholemeal flour products and other whole grains

These include compounds that feed the fertilized egg during the first few weeks of pregnancy, Ceylon or black tea has been shown to increase fertility. Milk products should be consumed in no more than two cups per day. Full-fat, organic milk and yogurt are recommended in moderation to boost fertility.

Foods to stay away from when trying to become pregnant:

- Caffeinated beverages and chocolate
- All diet beverages with artificial sweeteners

- Try honey or maple syrup instead of sugar, soda, and pasteurized juices, which are processed, refined, and artificial sugars.
- In addition to one or two cups of black tea each day, caffeine is known to have estrogen mimicking characteristics in soy products.

An increase in the occurrence of infertility throughout the globe has been linked to genetically modified foods' recognized ability to complicate conception. According to research, genetically modified foods may be one of the reasons why male sperm counts have decreased by as much as 40–50% globally since the 1970s. You may investigate genetically modified organisms (GMOs) on your own, however, the following is a quick summary of some of them:

Substantial amounts of red meat, bitter lemon, quinine, Sugar, and trans fats, meals without added fat, syrups made from starches like cornstarch and starch, and alcohol, cheese prepared with vegetable oil and rennet and GN meals made with soy that has been processed, certain genetically modified fruits, like papaya

A word on fat-free foods

Foods that are fat-free or low in fat often have a high sugar content and are extensively processed. Foods that are as near to their natural state as possible should be preferred. Because hormone production requires fat, a full-fat dairy diet, for instance, has been found in Harvard research to boost fertility.

Especially in males, alcohol may drastically impair fertility.

Drinking more reduces a woman's chance of becoming pregnant. Alcohol use, according to research, lowers the percentage of motile sperm, increases the amount of defective sperm, and lowers sperm count. The body's ability to absorb nutrients like zinc, one of the most crucial elements for male fertility, is also hampered by alcohol. Alcohol use is not recommended for women who are trying to become pregnant since it will interfere with their efforts to get their bodies in the best possible shape for conception. Women should significantly reduce or entirely stop drinking alcohol before attempting to conceive.

Whole foods are where you'll find the most taste, fiber, enzymes, and antioxidants. They don't include any extra sugar, fat, preservatives, tastes, or colors. The finest meals are straightforward, pure, and entire. Consuming carbohydrates gradually causes blood sugar levels to rise more gradually and with less vigor.

Consuming slow-digesting carbohydrates improves fertility, lowers insulin resistance, and regulates blood sugar. Examples of slow-releasing carbohydrates include beans, peas, lentils, whole grains, and the majority of vegetables.
The antioxidant and fiber content of plant-based foods such as fruits, vegetables,

legumes, nuts, seeds, and whole grains is substantial. A vegan or vegetarian diet that consists mostly of plants may also include small quantities of dairy, fish, meat, and other animal products.

Consume organic fruits and vegetables regularly. Wash your vegetables well before eating them, and avoid any that you suspect may have been sprayed with potentially harmful pesticides and herbicides that have been shown to reduce both male and female fertility. Organically cultivated fruits and vegetables have higher nutrients. Try buying at a farm stand or market instead of a supermarket!

Antioxidant-rich foods including fruits, vegetables, herbs, and spices are almost always organic. The oxidative stress and cellular inflammation associated with decreased fertility are lowered by these foods.

While reducing cellular inflammation, healthy fats and oils increase hormone sensitivity and function. Whole plant foods including coconuts, nuts, seeds, avocados, and fish are natural sources of them.

Dairy products that are advised for fertility include small amounts of plain, full-fat, live-culture yogurt and organic cheeses. Most reproductive issues may benefit greatly from a full-fat dairy diet, but dairy should be avoided by women who have endometriosis or PCOS since it might exacerbate these conditions. The hormone estrogen, which causes painful and heavy menstruation, cramps, diarrhea, nausea, and vomiting, is activated by prostaglandins, which are raised by dairy products. They might also agitate and upset the body's equilibrium.

Contrary to Chinese medicine, which stresses the elements of taste, texture, color, meal pairings, and manner that all contribute to its remarkable healing capacity, Western food philosophy often focuses on the qualities of food, such as vitamins and antioxidants. The need of slowing down and relaxing when eating is another theme in Chinese medicine.

As was previously said, it's important to eat food that is as close to its natural state as possible and to consume seasonal foods since they are often what the body requires at that particular time of year. Dedicate yourself to eating only when you are really hungry.

Studies have shown that women with the highest fertility rates and the lowest risk of ovulation problems are those who consume a plant-based, low glycemic index (GI), whole-food diet that includes at least one dish of high-fat dairy each day.

Foods were created by nature to aid in feeding and nourishing the body. The ability of the human body to repair, rebuild, and restore itself is astounding when it is provided with the optimum diet. This is highly good for improving fertility. A balanced diet may help lower the chance of miscarriage because of insulin resistance,

DNA damage from free radicals, and the caliber of the egg and sperm.

The kind of carbohydrates a person consumes has a big effect on their fertility. Carbohydrates regulate the amounts of insulin and blood sugar. When these levels are excessively high, ovulation is interfered with. High GI meals raise the possibility of ovulatory infertility and result in a sharp rise in insulin, which delivers an immediate boost to energy and is then followed by a depressing low.

Diets rich in slow, high-fiber carbohydrates (low GI meals), which help to boost fertility, often include whole grains, brown rice, legumes, and vegetables. Because they induce less of a spike in blood sugar after eating, low GI meals provide longer sensations of fullness, less blood sugar volatility, and longer-lasting energy. Low GI foods are linked to improved weight management, better physical performance, diabetes prevention and treatment, and mental stability. Pregnant women who consume a diet rich in these slow carbohydrates before becoming pregnant may avoid gestational diabetes, which is an increasing worry for them and their unborn children.

Including whole grains, dry beans and peas, vegetables, entire fruits, and other low and medium GI items in your diet may assist to encourage ovulation. Avoid eating foods with a high GI.

Examples of low GI foods are:

- Potatoes
- Sweet bread made with buckwheat
- Oat bran or pumpernickel
- Kidney beans
- Lentils
- Chickpeas quinoa
- Fruits and vegetables with barley
- Yogurt with whole milk

Foods that are high in GI include:

- Red potato
- Split peas
- Oats
- Popcorn
- Stout rice
- Couscous

- Brahmi rice bread made of granules
- Rash bread

High GI meals should be avoided while trying to become pregnant, such as:

- Potatoes
- White rice
- White bread
- Belgian waffles with French toast
- Almost all breakfast cereals, bagels\soda\sweets
- Sweet carbonated drinks
- French fries.

Additionally, it is possible to lower a food's GI by adding:

- Citric acid vinegar

- Oleic acid

- Mixing low-GI foods, such as beans and wild rice, with others that have medium or high GIs.

Focus on eating more legumes, healthy grains, and vegetables rather than sugary drinks and processed carbohydrates (breads, muffins, cakes, cookies).

CHAPTER FOUR

WATER IS NECESSARY, SO SIP AWAY

Make sure you drink enough water each day to equal at least half your body weight in ounces. Avoid drinking water from plastic bottles since some of the chemicals in plastics may lead to hormonal irregularities. Never drink water from a bottle that has been in a warm car to hydrate yourself! This is highly risky and maybe quite toxic, even if you are not trying to become pregnant. Your best alternatives are reverse osmosis and distilled water. Avoid consuming tap water since new research has shown that it is tainted with harmful agricultural chemicals. For other reproductive problems, there are even more specific diets to follow.

After starting your fertility diet, you should feel considerably better right away, but it takes some time for the body to respond and heal. For true, long-lasting effects on your general health and fertility, you must include a fertility diet into your lifestyle and everyday routine.

Dietary Program for Fertility

Food affects the body's capacity to generate hormones, fight free radicals, and store fat. Undoubtedly, a healthy diet may increase your fertility. The dietary recommendations listed below will aid with your infertility.

Detoxify

Eat only natural foods. You should avoid consuming any partly prepared or boxed meals since they can contain harmful ingredients.

The best option is to make meals from scratch, even if it may take some time. The items you choose shouldn't include artificial coloring, scent, preservatives, or flavorings. Make sure you choose organic vegetables. Pesticide residues and nitrates have the potential to interfere with hormone balance, which might be problematic for women who are trying to become pregnant.

The Importance of Fat in Fertility

Our brains are wired to believe that fat should be avoided. However, frequent use of some full-fat dairy products may benefit female fertility.

Some studies link animal lipids to improved ovarian function. According to Harvard University research, using full-fat dairy products significantly decreases the risk of infertility.

Colored food has a superior flavor

Yes, start making food selections based on color! Brightness and vibrancy are ideal.

Orange, yellow, and green foods should be a regular part of your diet. These product items include essential vitamins and minerals for wellness. They will also be abundant in antioxidants, which are essential for ridding the body of harmful free radicals.

Throw out the booze and coffee. Goodbye

You'll need to remove some of your favorites from your diet plan while also adding some new ones. It has coffee in it.

Although the reason why coffee harms fertility is difficult to pinpoint, specialists have come to the same conclusion. Even though one cup of coffee a day is not harmful, all caffeinated beverages should be avoided by women who are having problems becoming pregnant.

Alcohol adheres to the same rules. Several studies have shown a link between drinking and infertility. While the occasional glass of wine is OK, try to moderate your consumption.

Optimal Lipids And fatty fish

To promote health, full-fat dairy products should also be ingested together with fatty acids and unsaturated fats. Eating these meals will reduce the inflammatory response and increase your insulin sensitivity.

Salmon and other fatty fish are ideal. Increased consumption of avocados, raw almonds, sardines, and pumpkin seeds is recommended.

Some of the most all-encompassing and organic methods for accelerating the process of conception are only the beginning, and they don't even involve a fertility eating regimen.

Possibilities of a Fertility Diet

Healthy eating has always been emphasized by parents to their children as a means to boost their immune systems. But since we were the stubborn little children that we were, I'm sure that we all chose to eat junk food because it was more pleasurable. We were unaware that maturing can have a detrimental effect on our reproductive system. Yes, it is conceivable that the body won't be able to produce healthy eggs or sperm, which is essential for maintaining the pregnancy, as a consequence of hormonal changes. By following a diet that is nutrient-dense enough for fertility, you may speed up the process of becoming pregnant.

Because infertility is a serious problem for today's youth as a result of the growth of science through generations, more individuals are becoming experts in a variety of fields to help couples who want to start families. A fertility diet may also be quite helpful since it may regulate the body's hormone levels. Increase your intake of nutrient-dense meals that are rich in calcium, vitamins, and minerals. You should eat a lot of green and leafy vegetables in addition to fruits that serve as antioxidants.

When following a fertility diet, dietitians advise against dangerous habits including smoking, drinking, using drugs, and staying up late. You must keep a disciplined lifestyle since all of these factors might cause conception to be delayed. Your body and mind need enough sleep to be able to adjust to the various changes that your body may go through. You could also be given medication along with all of these protective steps. To have a speedier and more pleasurable pregnancy, please remember to take them as directed.

And also your male counterpart because he too may experience infertility, it is imperative that your male counterpart maintains a healthy diet. Your fertility diet plan will include a list of items to avoid as well as fruits and vegetables that both men and women should eat. Even the benefits will be covered so you can see why a particular vegetable has been suggested to you. Lean meats will also be a part of this diet because fish is abundant in omega-3 fatty acids and chicken is a good source of protein. Because your body will be working hard while receiving fertility medicine or any other sort of fertility therapy, you must eat healthily.

A reproductive diet plan includes mostly 100% safe organic items, whether or not it uses Chinese supplements. Eating fresh meals and correctly preparing them can be quite beneficial to us. However, the results can be much improved if we are fully aware of what to avoid eating and drinking.

Purified water. All fertility diet regimens will warn you about the health concerns that drinking tap water without filtering it can expose you to and will advise you to do so using any readily available devices in your location. Whether you drink the water straight up or use it to cook with, you'll feel safer knowing that it has been fully filtered.

Dangerous fats. Modern diet specialists place tremendous emphasis on the type and amount of fat that we ingest. If you want to ensure a healthy diet and increase fertility, you must stay away from trans fats, which are frequently found in chips, fries, chocolate, biscuits, doughnuts, and other takeaway meals. animals' production of estrogens. Another category of foods that we must stay away from in a perfect fertility diet plan is anything that can upset our hormonal balance. One of the numerous issues caused by the hormones found in cow's milk is infertility.

Canned food. Even the reproductive diet components much less the healthy diet components must not contain any preservatives. Stick to fresh fruits and vegetables and home-cooked meals if you want to maintain your body healthy and capable of becoming pregnant.

1. A good fertility diet will not include anything that makes you feel uncomfortable. Allergies can threaten the development of an embryo in a mother who may have become pregnant easily and will surely have an impact on a woman who is not yet pregnant. As such, you should avoid

allergens and take care of any allergies you may already have (if any).

Coffee and Alcohol. You will notice that the recipes for the fertility diet do not contain any alcohol or coffee. These two popular drinks should be avoided if you want to increase your fertility. They have a history of causing miscarriages and may even impair your immune system.

CHAPTER FIVE

FOOD THAT AID IN WOMEN'S FERTILITY

Diet has a significant impact on the preconception process. You should regularly include these foods in your diet if you're trying to get pregnant because it's believed that they boost fertility. You are not required to limit yourself to delectable food when trying to get pregnant. Reality is quite the opposite.

Women can increase their fertility by eating the foods listed below:

Fruit and vegetable freshness.
Fruits and vegetables should also be consumed by those who are trying to conceive. Fruits and vegetables provide vital vitamins, nutrients, and antioxidants that promote overall health, including reproductive health. Green leafy vegetables and citrus fruits, such as strawberries and oranges, are also mentioned as excellent sources of folate. Folate is an essential element that helps prevent birth abnormalities.

Grain total. You can consume large amounts of only complex carbohydrates. Complex carbohydrates do not affect your insulin or blood sugar levels in the same way that refined carbohydrates, such as those found in white bread and sugar, do. Everything that makes insulin work more effectively improves fertility. Among the foods that are rich sources of complex carbohydrates are whole grains like oats, whole grain loaves of bread, stone ground cornmeal, and brown rice.

Products Produced using Full-Fat Dairy. Contrary to popular belief, dairy products with extra fat have been shown to boost fertility. According to studies, women who consumed dairy products in their entirety had fewer ovulation problems than those who consumed dairy products with little to no fat. To increase your chances of becoming pregnant, consume whole milk, full-fat yogurt, or ice cream (delicious!).

Foods High in Vitamin Zn. Zinc must be consumed by women who are trying to get pregnant. Studies have shown that oysters, which are rich in zinc, improve a woman's fertility. Zinc aids in the production of high-quality eggs and assists in maintaining a regular menstrual cycle. Zinc can be found in abundance in

- Lean meat
- Eggs
- Chicken
- Fish
- Wheat germ
- Sunflower seeds
- Whole grains

- Oats
- Legumes

Food Sources of Vitamins C and E

Vitamins C and E are powerful antioxidants that assist in repairing the body from the damage brought on by free radicals. Furthermore, it's believed that combining these two vitamins may increase ovulation and increase fertility in women who are infertile for unknown reasons. Vitamin C-rich foods include citrus fruits, mangos, cherries, strawberries, grapes, cantaloupe, pineapples, kiwi, tomatoes, asparagus, and spinach. Foods high in vitamin E include whole grains, nuts, seeds, avocados, wheat germ, molasses, eggs, organ meats, and products made from organ meats.

Diet for both men's and women's fertility

One of the most important traits that all humans value highly is their capacity for procreation. Once you've settled down in life, both sexes enjoy procreating and having children. There's nothing wrong with that, but it just goes to show how important it is to eat right to increase your chances of getting pregnant. You must include particular foods in your diet because a fertility diet is essential for increasing your productivity at all times.

That way, you can be sure your children will be strong and healthy. Please read the brief guidelines I've provided below to make sure you can duplicate them without any problems. Both the male and female reproductive systems are essential to pregnancy. To put it another way, both sexes must be in good health and, more importantly, must consume healthfully because reproduction requires both.

Making sure your diet is rich in antioxidants is the first thing you should do if you're a man. These antioxidants increase fertility by lowering oxidative damage to male sperm. If you didn't know, one of the most important diets for fertility that applies to both men and women emphasizes eating foods high in iron. It's because this essential element, which provides the body with the necessary strength, is so important.

You can eat things like

- Beans
- Chicken
- Spinach
- Meat
- A small amount of fish as part of a healthy diet.

Both diets, vegetarian or not, are catered to, as you can see from the list above. You can also increase your fertility by including fruits and vegetables in your diet. This type of fertility diet is essential, especially for men. As was mentioned earlier, they offer vitamins and antioxidants that increase male fertility.

Furthermore, it's important to maintain an active lifestyle since when you live a boring, inactive life, your body doesn't receive any exercise. When you don't exercise regularly, your reproductive system doesn't work as effectively. As a result, be careful to maintain a healthy weight and engage in regular exercise. When you are actively trying to become pregnant, you should cut off coffee. Caffeine's primary drawback is its decreased ability to provide blood to the uterus.

If you adhere to the recommended fertility diet, you will become pregnant at the right time.

Beverages to Have

Other women struggle far less than others to conceive, yet some have less trouble. The following "rules" must be followed by women to become pregnant, according to fertility experts:

It is advised to engage in regular exercise, keep a healthy weight, let go of stress, unwind, and consume a diet rich in foods that support fertility.

- Refrain from consuming coffee, alcoholic beverages, and smoking.
- Time sexual activity to coincide with a woman's reproductive periods.
- Antioxidants
- Vitamin C

- Folic acid
- Selenium
- Zinc
- Omega-3 fatty acids
- Vitamin B complex
- Vitamin D
- Folic acid.

The body's capacity to control hormones and the health of the female reproductive system are supported by these vitamins and minerals. While it is possible to buy each of these vitamins and minerals individually, it is more practical to buy prenatal multivitamins or fertility-boosting supplements from herbal stores that include most or all of the aforementioned vitamins and minerals in a single tablet or capsule of course, because these foods are excellent sources of vitamins and minerals, it is a great idea to eat fresh produce as regularly as you can.

In addition to eating a varied, healthy, and well-balanced diet, there are a few things that you should try to eat Naturally, a key factor in enhancing female fertility is good nutrition, just as enhancing male fertility requires good nutrition. The nutrients that boost both male and female fertility are not all equal, however. Women who eat foods rich in the following nutrients have the highest chance of becoming pregnant:

most days.

Fatty fish include essential fatty acids (EFAs) including omega 3 and 6.

Avocados contain a lot of vitamin E.

Chilies include vitamin C, which helps to relieve tension and release endorphins.

The most important nutrient for fertility is zinc, which may be found in oysters.

Spinach contains significant amounts of iron, folic acid, and vitamin C.

Iron and vitamin B12 are abundant in lean red meat.

In honey, there are several minerals and amino acids.

Garlic, which is known to help increase low sperm counts, also contains selenium and vitamin B6.

In conclusion: So, if you frequently consume foods that aid in conception, particularly if you've been trying to become pregnant for a long time, you could find that you ultimately get pregnant.